Aerobic Exercise: Great Routines to Foster Healthy Living

Fitness Tips on Effective Aerobic Routines

By: Jana Duncan

9781630225681

TABLE OF CONTENTS

PUBLISHERS NOTES

Speedy Publishing LLC

40 E. Main St., #1156

Newark, DE 19711

www.speedypublishing.co

Cover Artwork: 24 Hr. Designs Ltd.

Editing: Speedy Publishing LLC

Book design: Speedy Publishing LLC

ISBN: 9781630225681

This is a reprint book.

DISCLAIMER

This publication is intended to provide helpful and informative material. It is not intended to diagnose, treat, cure, or prevent any health problem or condition, nor is intended to replace the advice of a physician. No action should be taken solely on the contents of this book. Always consult your physician or qualified health-care professional on any matters regarding your health and before adopting any suggestions in this book or drawing inferences from it.

The author and publisher specifically disclaim all responsibility for any liability, loss or risk, personal or otherwise, which is incurred as a consequence, directly or indirectly, from the use or application of any contents of this book.

Any and all product names referenced within this book are the trademarks of their respective owners. None of these owners have sponsored, authorized, endorsed, or approved this book.

Always read all information provided by the manufacturers' product labels before using their products. The author and publisher are not responsible for claims made by manufacturers.

DEDICATION

This one is for you as well, Rick and Julie. Stick with the game plan and you'll start seeing results.

INTRODUCTION

Aerobics is a form of exercise that is repetitive and full of rhythmic motion.

If you really want to get your body in shape, aerobics is the way to go. It is one of the most popular exercise formats that you can use to get flexible and increase the strength in your muscles.

Aerobics will also help you to increase your metabolism and have more energy. There are several celebrity trainers that use aerobic workouts and have videos that people can purchase and follow along at home.

When you are doing aerobic exercises, you are using your major muscle groups which help to increase your heart rates. When you are doing aerobics on a regular basis, your body will able to use more oxygen and have more energy. Your heart will be stronger and your lungs will be optimized.

In order to perform aerobic exercises, you need to have enough oxygen so that you can breathe properly. There are different kinds of aerobic exercises. The most common and popular ones are walking, running, swimming and bicycling. There is also step aerobics, which can be done at home or joining a class at the health club.

Aerobics is a great way to tone and strengthen your body. Your lungs are strengthened as you breathe and your heart muscle gets larger. The blood in your system won't need a lot to pump to your heart.

Aerobic Exercise: Great Routines to Foster Healthy Living

This also helps your blood circulation and keeps your blood pressure level. Your red blood cell count will increase and your muscles will have more fat storage and more carbs. This will help you have more energy which gives you a longer period of time to do aerobics.

Aerobics is one of the easiest ways that you can exercise in order to get fit. It can help you lose weight and eliminate stress. People can do aerobic exercises at least three to four times a week for at least 30 minutes a day starting out. Then as they get more energy, they can increase the time limit.

Don't push yourself to the place that you want to be. Take your time when you are doing aerobic exercise. If you start out overdoing it, you can hurt your joints and muscles.

Before you start your workout, you should always warm up with stretching for about 10 minutes so that your muscles will not be stiff when you are ready to start. After you have finished, cool down with about 10 minutes of stretching.

If you are not sure about doing aerobic exercises, get with your physician for further consultation.

One of the main purposes for aerobics is that it can be used to burn a lot of fat from your body. You need to work most in the area where you need to get rid of a lot of fat.

Walking, running and riding a bike are some of the best ways to burn the fat from your body. You can do any of these exercises in moderation.

Aerobics can only be effective for you if you are doing it at certain times. It can be done in the morning before you eat or any time that you can fit in during the evening.

Jana Duncan

In the morning before eating – make sure that you have drunk at least 24 ounces of water before you start. This will help you from becoming dehydrated. Doing aerobics in the morning will help you to burn more body fat than any other time during the day. There is nothing in your body to burn so aerobics affects where the fat is stored to retrieve energy that is needed to get you moving.

CHAPTER 1- OTHER BENEFITS OF AEROBIC ACTIVITY

Aerobics helps to improve the cardio respiratory endurance of an individual.

Lungs – Doing aerobics can affect your lungs to where the muscles that are used to breathe gain more strength. If you have any chronic illnesses, such as bronchitis or asthma, aerobics can help with that as well. These illnesses, along with emphysema, will help you to breathe better. Aerobics also helps you to gain an advantage with oxygen for your lungs.

Heart – If you do aerobics at least three times every week, your heart rate will increase. Your heart will also be able to pump additional blood into your body. Your muscles will get oxygen at a quicker rate.

Muscles – Your muscles will gain more strength when you do aerobics. They also get larger and your body will become leaner because you will have more muscle mass. Your muscles will also increase in body fat so that you will have more energy. Your metabolism will increase due to the lean muscle, which results in you losing more weight.

Burn calories - Since aerobics is a fat burning exercise, you will burn more calories quickly. The more fat that you burn, the more weight that you will lose; hence the loss of calories.

CHAPTER 2- DOING AEROBICS AT HOME

There are many forms of aerobic exercise and the tops ones are aerobic dance, walking, cycling, running, swimming and cross-country skiing.

If taking an aerobics class is out of your budget, then you can do them at home. In fact, it's probably easier to do because you can be more relaxed and you don't have to use gas to go anywhere. The exercises can be done in the comfort of your own home. It does not matter how you look because no one will see you.

Aerobic is an easy exercise routine to start out at home. If you are one of those people who have not worked out in a while and your body is not looking its best, doing aerobics at home can help you from being embarrassed in front of others. Once you get into shape, you can venture outside to take some classes.

Just because you are doing aerobics at home does not mean that you won't get the same benefits that you would if you were in a class. You would still be able to enhance your health and get your heart and lungs strong, lose weight and be able to reduce stress.

Even though you are at home, you should do aerobics exercises starting at three times a week, 30 minutes a day and work your way up. You can increase the intensity of your sessions as you feel you are ready.

You can use a treadmill to work out. You can probably one that is one sale. Treadmills don't cost a lot either.

You can also use aerobic exercise videos to get you started. You may have to watch it once or twice to get the hang of what's going on. There is step aerobics, dancing, kickboxing and other different

Aerobic Exercise: Great Routines to Foster Healthy Living
styles of aerobics. Start out at the level that you feel most comfortable with. For many people, that would be the beginning level.

Videos can be bought from retailers such as Wal-Mart or Target. Or if you don't want to go out, you can order them online. They videos usually come in a series, so you would get the benefit of doing several different aerobic exercises.

If you are one of those people that is not disciplined enough to do this on your own, see if you can get a partner to join you. It could be your spouse, a friend or your children, provided that they are old enough.

Having a partner can help you with that support that you need to keep going when you want to quit. Even if you're not thinking about quitting, a partner can help you to the next level.

Try and do your aerobic exercises when there aren't other people around. That way you won't be interrupted.

CHAPTER 3- STEP AEROBICS

Aerobics has been a popular form of exercise since the 1960's.

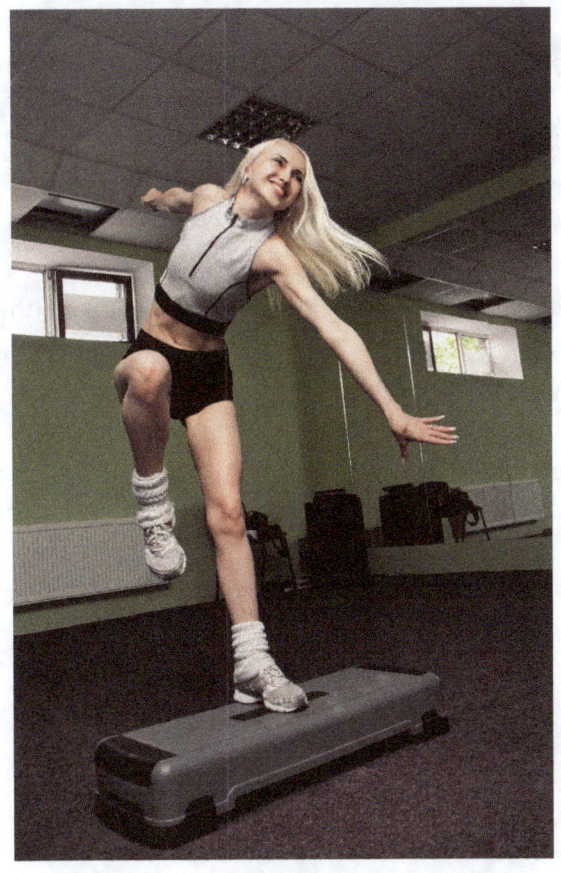

This style of aerobics uses a platform that is elevated. This aerobics is very popular with a lot of people. You will exercise with music that has a fast beat along with steps that coordinate with the beats. You will find this kind of aerobics exercise performed at health clubs and gyms as a class. However, you can purchase a step aerobics package and do it on your own at home.

The platform raises no more than a foot off the ground. The sessions are usually no longer than an hour. However, there are some half-hour sessions as well. How it works is you will step on and off of the platform according to the beat of the music. There are different ways of stepping where you have to use the platform.

You can burn calories using step aerobics. Your muscles will also get strong and your metabolism will increase. The oxygen in your body will increase. Your heart will beat faster and build up stamina. Once your heart gets up to speed, more blood will be able to flow to your body.

This is a low impact exercise. You have to make sure that you are doing it right, otherwise you could hurt your knees and joints. Whether you are following a video or an instructor, pay attention to every step. You should be wearing shoes that are comfortable and made to perform exercises of this kind. They should have rubber on the bottom that is not slippery.

If you have never done step aerobics before, please consult with your physician prior to starting.

Chapter 4- How To Get Ready For Step Aerobics

The body gets more oxygen rich blood from aerobic exercise.

Using these precautions before you start your step aerobics workout will help you to get the best out of it. It will also help prevent injuries that can be inflicted if you don't do it correctly.

Before you start, make sure that you are in good enough shape to start this aerobic exercise. Otherwise, you will find yourself out of breath before you get into it good enough.

Your foot should be on the step. It should be the entire foot, not part of it. You need to be able to balance well when you are stepping on and off. If you don't you could lose your balance and possibly fall or injure yourself. This is crucial if you are stepping to fast music.

The knees should measure up over your ankles. Don't do lunges as you are stepping up on to the platform. You want to make sure that the knee stays over the ankle each time you step up.

Only use so many risers with the step. Two or three risers should be the recommended amount, depending on your height. The stepper needs to be comfortable enough where you won't endure stress with your back and your knees.

Keep a straight posture as you step up and down. Do not bend your back or hips forward. When you are doing step aerobics, skip the hand or ankle weights. Using weights while you are stepping can cause injuries to your knees, shoulders and ankles. You are already

Aerobic Exercise: Great Routines to Foster Healthy Living
moving fast and having weights is an extra burden that can stress
out the joints.

CHAPTER 5- RUNNING

Running does help to reduce the strain in the heart.

Running is one of the best and cost effective ways to get fit. This aerobic exercise can benefit young and old people. When you run, you are doing so at a measured pace. It's faster than a jog, but slower than a complete run. You should run in moderation and don't look to do a hard run. A hard run is not considered aerobic exercising.

Depending on how you function during the day, you can choose to run in the morning or in the afternoons or evening. Everyone does not respond the same when it comes to running.

Before you start, you would have to check out the weather and the environment you would be doing this in. All places are different and there may be some that are not conducive for running. So check out the area before you decide to commit.

You have to prepare yourself for the weather at hand. If it's cool, you will need clothing that will keep your warm. It it's warm, you will need clothing that will keep you cool. You will also need the right kind of shoes to wear when you start running. You will need to be comfortable so that you can get the best fitness workout.

CHAPTER 6- WHERE TO GO RUNNING

A study done on fifty thousand US Air Force personnel led to the start of aerobics. This study was conducted by Major Kenneth H. Cooper

There are different places where you can go running. You can do it in your neighborhood, on a park trail, or anywhere that you feel safe doing this. Make sure that you are running on flat ground or a flat surface.

Don't take the chance running on slopes that are difficult, rough areas or slippery areas. There's a greater chance that you would get injured. The last thing that you need is a sprained ankle or a pulled muscle.

If you are more experienced, there are some slopes and inclines that are made for running. Check out the areas first before you commit to running. Stay near areas where you can get immediate help if needed.

The area where you will be running should not have any obstacles. You need to be free to run so that you can stay on course.

If you find areas where you can run, but they are far away from where you live, find alternative places that are closer and just as good. There may be times when you will not be able to go to those far away spots when you want to.

It's not a bad idea to have a running buddy run with you. They can give you great support.

Jana Duncan

Always try to go to an area where there are not a lot of other runners. This can throw off your exercise regimen and make you not want to run.

CHAPTER 7- WARMING UP

Warming up before exercising helps to stretch the muscles properly and reduce the possibility of injury.

There's no doubt—you must warm up before you start running. Make it a habit every time you run to warm up. It is an important part of your aerobic exercise. You can prevent unnecessary injuries. Many sports athletes know that they have to do this before every game or else they can risk being injured. You are no different in that aspect. Your muscles need to be loose before you start moving.

You can warm up your muscles for about 10 – 15 minutes and make them flexible. If your muscles are cold and you don't warm them up, you will not get the output that you desire. You could also pull a muscle in the process.

You can do light cardiovascular exercises in order for the blood to flow through your body. Light jogging is another way that you can warm up before you start running. Whatever you use for warm up exercises, they should be low impact and light, such as lunges.

Don't rest after you have warmed up. Do some stretches so that you will keep your momentum going. You want to be ready to run right after you're finished. Don't overstretch your joints and muscles or you could cause injury to those areas.

Then you can start running and get into your exercise.

CHAPTER 8- HYDRATION

During exercise, it is essential to keep hydrated as lots of liquid get lost through sweat.

It's important to stay hydrated while before and during your running exercise. This can prevent you from suffering heat related illnesses. If you don't drink enough, you can get tired, uncoordinated and your muscles can start to cramp. You can also pass out, especially in warm weather.

You can also experience a heatstroke, exhaustion from the heat. When you are running, you need to know how much you are drinking through the entire process.

Prior to you running, you should drink at least 24 ounces of water. This should be done at least an hour before you start. If not water, drink something that does not contain caffeine. Twenty-four ounces of water should be enough to get you started. Having more than that can stop your exercise regimen and force you to go to the bathroom.

While you are running, drink at least eight ounces of fluids that don't contain caffeine. This should be done at least every 20 minutes. If you are running for more than an hour and a half, include a sports drink to replenish sodium and minerals.

Have a water bottle or something similar that you can carry your fluids in during your running exercise. This is for those who don't have access to water on their route while they are running.

After you have finished running, you will need to replenish the fluids that you sweated during your exercise. Check the color of your urine afterwards. If the color is dark yellow, drink more fluids. Your urine should be a light yellow.

These tips will help you to stay hydrated and able to run the course. The last thing you need is to pass out while you are out and about.

CHAPTER 9- RUNNING TIPS

Always ensure that the appropriate shoes are worn for running to prevent injury.

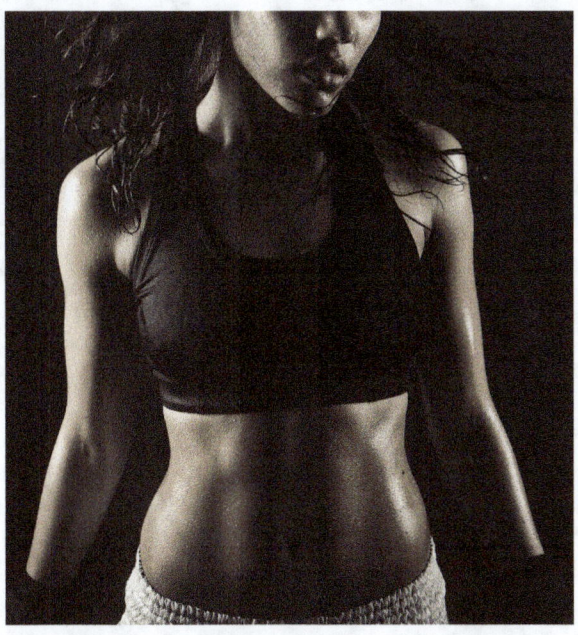

When running, you can't just do it any kind of way. There are things that you need to know in order to have an effective workout.

• When you are running, don't look at your feet. You need to look ahead because you need to see what's coming in the event you need to get out of the way of danger.

• When you land, use the center of your foot and go to the front of your toes. Don't land on your toes. If you do, you will get tired quickly. You can also injure your shin and cause tightness in your calves. Don't land on your heels because you can get injured.

• Keep your hands at your waist. Use a 90 degree angle for your arms. You get tired quicker if your hands are up by your chest. Your shoulders and neck will tighten.

• Keep your hands relaxed. They can be cupped as though you were holding something. Your fists should not be clenched because it can tighten your shoulders and arms.

• While you are running, keep our back straight and your head up. Take a look at your posture to see that everything is in place. Poke out your chest when you are feeling slumped over.

• Keep your shoulders in a square position and make sure they are relaxed. They should not be stiff or hunched. Don't bring your shoulders too far to the front. Your chest can tighten and you won't be able to breathe well.

• Swing your shoulders towards the front and back using the joints from your shoulders.

CHAPTER 10- BOUNCING

Running properly will guarantee a great workout. Bouncing will use up excess energy.

As you run, try to avoid bouncing. If you move up and down too much, you have used up energy that you did not need to use. The lower portion of your body can be affected by this movement. The higher up you are the more shock that is sucked in as you land on the ground. This results in you and your legs getting tired faster than they need to be.

In order to cut the bouncing down to a bare minimum, do some light running and when you land, land on your feet softly. Your feet should be low to the ground level and using brief strides. Your arms should still be at a 90 degree angle and bent. When you swing them, the swing should be shorter and lower.

Don't run on your toes. Running on your toes can contribute to bouncing.

Keep a Log

In order to keep up with your progress, have a log where you can write down the information. Keeping up with this log will help you to see where you are and where you could be. It can be considered as a motivational tool to keep you going. Make sure to keep up with all dates, times and miles. Also, write some comments about that day's exercise.

Start Out Slow

When you start running, don't try to be like the NASCAR drivers and take off running. Start off slow and work your way up. Starting out fast does nothing for you except giving you exhaustion and soreness that you don't need. When you do too much in the beginning, you can also incur unnecessary injuries. Do everything gradually and you will get to your destination. Running will be more fun to you if you don't get ahead of yourself, ending up with stresses and injuries.

Weather

If you are used to running whether it's hot or cold, make sure that you are properly dressed. Having the right clothing makes a difference when you are exercising. You need to feel comfortable while you are running. If the weather is so rough where you can't do it outside, then find an inside gym where they have running facilities.

Running For Fun

Even though you are running to get fit, don't make it as though it's such a dreadful chore. You want to have fun and be able to release some steam from people or events that rattled you. You also want to improve your health. If you are running outdoors, take in some of the scenery that you would otherwise may not get to see.

CHAPTER 11- WALKING

Walking is a great form of aerobic exercise for those who have joint problems or who should not be doing strenuous forms of exercise.

Walking is one of the easiest aerobics that you can do. Not only does it not cost you anything, but to get up and go, anyone can do it. Whether the pace is slow or fast, walking is good for everyone.

It only takes 30 minutes a day to complete an effective walking workout. You can start walking three days a week and produce some results. Once you get accustomed to walking, it will be time to do it with more intensity.

Aerobic walking helps to increase your heart and breathing rate. When you start walking every day, you will start to get more fit. You will also be able to avoid some health risks such as cancer, heart ailments and diabetes.

Other benefits of aerobic walking include:

- Having control of your weight
- Muscular fitness
- Being able to balance your body
- Lowers blood pressure
- Less chance of having a stroke or other kinds of cancer

Being injured by walking is not common. It is one of the safest, if not the safest aerobic exercise that everyone can do.

It is recommended that you do at least two and a half hours of aerobic activity every week. That means you can do aerobic walking for 30 minutes a day, five days a week. Even though it may not start out that way, you will eventually work your way up to that point.

Start out by determining how many times a week you will do the aerobic walking. You will need to know how long you will do it for each day that you go out. If you are rusty and have not walked in a while, take your time when you start out.

Some people may do exercises in 10 minute intervals, which is a great idea for the ones who haven't been exercising in a while. Gradually, you will add more time and intensity to your walk. The key is to start out gradually and don't rush to get to the next level.

Before you start, see your physician to get approval for doing this. Not having walked in a while may cause some issues if you don't know what you are doing. Unless you have some type of physical limitations, your physician will probably give the green light.

CHAPTER 12- WALKING EQUIPMENT AND ACCESSORIES

Though aerobics is important, careful consideration has to be put into the gear that is used as well for both comfort and safety.

In order to enhance your aerobic walking exercises, you will need:

Apparel – Whatever your wear should be comfortable and lightweight. You don't want to wear anything tight where your skin cannot breathe. Clothes that are made from cotton are good to wear.

If you are a night walker, wear light clothing and use reflective tape if you are sharing the road with vehicles. They will be able to see you. Not too many people walk at night, but if you do, have a partner. It's dangerous to walk by yourself when it's dark.

Walking shoes – When you start walking, you want to feel comfortable. Your walking shoes should be lightweight and durable. Get a pair that have a round heel and are breathable. Water resistant shoes are good if you will be walking in various kinds of weather.

Using a pedometer will help you to measure your walking distance. It's easy to use. You just program it and attach it to your belt or waistband. Once you have finished walking, you will know how long you have walked for that time period.

While you are walking, you should find out what you target heart rate is. It's important to know that so that you can either increase or decrease how fast you are walking. There are several accessories you can use for that purpose:

- Ankle weights
- Hand weights
- Wrist weights

In order to calculate your heart rate, you would take your age and remove that number from 220. Then you would take the difference and multiply it by the percentage you are looking to shoot for.

Increasing Aerobic Walking

The more that you walk,, the more that you will get fit. So this means you will have to eventually start walking every day. Make it a habit and gradually work your way up to that point.

Stick with the 150 minutes or so per week. As you continue at that pace, you can work your way up to 45 minutes or an hour per week.

Keep up with your progress. Take daily readings of your aerobic walks. You will see how far you have come since you started. Once you see your numbers looking the same, you will know that it is time to make some adjustments to your fitness routine.

Once you start making strides, reward yourself. Some people go out to eat when they have reached an achievement. Some say you should skip the food. If you're not careful, you can overeat or eat the wrong foods. More rewarding things that you can do is go shopping for yourself, going to a movie, or getting your nails done or a massage. These are things that are worthy of rewards.

CHAPTER 13- HOW TO GET MORE BENEFIT FROM YOUR AEROBIC WALKS

Using weight while walking will help to increase overall stamina and endurance.

Add more distance to your walking routine. If you walk more, your heart and breathing rate will increase tremendously.

Add more days to your walk. When you get accustomed to walking three days a week, step it up to four or five days. Once you get accustomed to that, step it up to six or seven days.

Start walking faster. You will get more benefits from doing that. You will also gain more speed and be able to walk for longer periods.

You can use hand weights during your aerobic walking. You can start off by using ½ pound weights. Using weights can help you to burn calories while walking at the same time. Once you get used to those, increase the weight size.

You can also use ankle weights. Ankle weights are designed for your legs. They help to provide increased strength to your leg muscles. They also work to sculpt and tone your muscles along with burning calories. You will get a lot of benefit of using them while you are walking.

Include a short run in the middle of your aerobic walking. Start out running with about 100 steps or so. When you run, your heart rate will increase and your breathing will be faster. After seven days, increase the steps by another 100. Doing this can help you to get out of the same walking routine every day. It's always good to add a twist in your exercise so that you won't feel bored.

Eventually, you may want to have a change of scenery. Make some changes and walk different routes. If you can walk in your neighborhood, do that. If there is a nearby park, go there. Walking trails are always great places to do your exercise.

Don't continue to walk the same distance. There will be some days where you can have shorter walks and on other days have longer walks.

If you can deal with inclines, try walking on some hills. Doing this can be a challenge; so make sure that you are ready for it. Alternate between hills and flat ground from time to time.

You can also listen to music while you are walking. If not music, then you can listen to audio books. They can put your mind at ease. However, if you decide to do this, be sure to be aware of your surroundings. You may not be able to hear or see everything that is going on around you because your focused on listening to the audio.

Aerobic walking can be more fun if you have a buddy to go with you. Get a friend, neighbor or relative to join you. Having someone go with you can give you that motivation and push that you need to go forward. Not everyone can get pumped to exercise on their own.

During inclement weather, find an indoor facility such as a recreational center, shopping mall or if you have a treadmill at home, you can use that.

The sooner you start your aerobic walking, the sooner you can start getting fit. Once you start walking every day, keep going. Don't

Jana Duncan
stop walking for a period of time unless you have become ill where you can't do it at the time. When you get better, start back again and don't give up!

CHAPTER 14- BICYCLING (OR CYCLING)

Cycling is a high intensity form of aerobic exercise which helps to burn excess calories.

You can get several benefits from cycling. Not only will you be able to see the sights from the outside and get some fresh air, but you can also get fit. In addition to that, you will burn calories and fat.

Riding a bicycle is a great way to enhance your cardiovascular system. It also allows you not to deal with the pollution coming from other vehicles.

On a bicycle, when you are going uphill and riding at a high intensity, you will be able to gain muscle and burn fat from your body. Your small and large muscles will develop more and get even stronger. When your muscles get more developed, your body will look fit, lean and strong.

This aerobic exercise can also increase your metabolism. You will burn more calories when your metabolism is higher. Even after you have finished for the day, you will still burn more calories.

The core of your body will gain strength, including the muscles in the back and your abdomen. With that, bicycling helps you to have good posture and be able for your body to have a balance.

This is good for activities and tasks that require the weight of your back. Bicycling can help you to increase the capacity of your aerobics, reduce risks of certain illnesses, such as blood pressure, cholesterol and cancer.

Riding a bicycle on a regular basis can help your muscles to get oxygen easier. So when you are doing strenuous tasks or exercises, you won't feel long winded.

There are people who ride bicycles that use them to increase their cardiovascular system. If you are one of those who have a crippling ailment such as arthritis, you may not be able to do activities because of your knees. While toning the leg muscles, bicycling is also used to tone the backside.

There are people who will a stationary bicycle, but that does not help as much as one where you can ride around the park and around town for your fitness workout. When you are using one where you can move around more, you can shift your weight to your legs. You have to be careful that you don't overdo it for fear of damaging your knees.

There is an increase in people that are bicycling in order to stay fit. Because they are concerned about their health and how they look, this aerobic exercise has emerged as one of the more popular activities that people like and want to do. Plus, since you don't use gas, there's no reason why you can get fit and burn calories with a bicycle.

Cycling outdoors is good to do when:

- The weather is presentable
- If you have time to ride your bike
- If you can ride on a cycle path
- If you like to ride outdoors
- If you don't mind the vehicles and possible traffic

You can also go cycling on tracks, forests and beaches. Whatever way that suits you should be ok, as long as you are getting in a fitness workout.

- The height of the seat should be comfortable and high enough for you. If it's too low, let it up. If it's too high, let it down.
- Check the handle bars to make sure that they care comfortable enough for you and that you can reach them.
- Your seat should also be comfortable enough for you to sit down.

How to Start Riding Your Bicycle

Just because people own a bicycle does not mean that they know how to get started riding it. It is not difficult to get started on your journey to aerobic fitness.

Start out with short rides. Don't overdo it or overwhelm yourself for trying to break a record by going for longer trips. Starting out, shoot for at least an hour's ride up to 15 miles. Of course, you can do less than that, depending on your strength.

It's easier to start riding your bike in the park. While you're riding, you can go sightseeing at the same time. You will see areas that you had not seen before or just passed by without giving it a second look.

Once you start, you won't want to stop. This is a great way of getting a workout while being able to see lovely views on the outside.

CHAPTER 15- INJURIES AND HOW TO PREVENT THEM

Injuries can result from failure to warm up properly or from doing the exercise incorrectly.

Some people think of cycling as dangerous. That's because some of the bicyclists may not adhere to the road rules and can incur injuries.

One thing that you must do when you are on a bicycle is to wear a helmet. You want your head to be protected in the event of an accident. The brain is very delicate and once it gets injured, the recovery process could be lengthy.

It is very common to find out that bicycle injuries can affect your knees. The knee injuries can affect anyone that rides a bicycle.

Other bicycle injuries can be caused by:

- Not being prepared to ride for long stretches
- The gear you using is too high for where you are riding
- You are not fitting on bicycle correctly and the saddle is not adjusted for your height
- Trying to ride too many inclines in the beginning stages of riding your bike

Make sure that the height of your saddle on the bicycle is not too high when you are riding. It should be at a height where you are comfortable as you use your pedals. If you are too high on the saddle, you can experience knee pain at the posterior. The height of the saddle should not be too low, either. The knee's anterior will be affected.

The saddle should be fitted correctly so that you can sit on it right. If it is not, your muscles could go out of balance. To avoid an injury where you overuse your muscles while riding, set the saddle at an angle between 25 – 35 degrees.

If the ride is uncomfortable for you, then you won't be able to get very far with your aerobic bicycling. You can end up with other "overuse" injuries by overdoing it on the bicycle.

- Chronic nerve damage – riding you bike for long periods of time without resting
- Palm damage, carpal tunnel syndrome – overuse of bike riding
- Bicycle seat neuropathy – numbness, pain in the groin area; can lead to erectile or sexual dysfunction.

Chapter 16- How Bicycling Can Help You

Based on the level of fitness of the individual, bicycling can range from moderate to intense.

Once you start cycling at least four times a week, your body will start to look different. You will look more fit and toned than you ever have before. You will start to feel different and have a better outlook on life. You don't have to overdo it by riding on your bike for long periods of time. Up to a half hour several days a week will help you out a lot.

Once you get used to riding on a bicycle, you can increase the intensity and how long you are going to ride. You will be able to burn plenty of calories once it's all said and done. During this process, your body will still be intact. Even if you are training for a race, bicycle exercise is a great way to get in shape. So when that day comes, you will be ready to roll.

There are plenty of trails where you are allowed to ride your bicycle. You will be able to get in a nice aerobic workout unless the weather turns bad. Bicycling is a great fitness workout and can benefit your entire body.

You don't have to be a professional to ride on a bicycle in order to get in shape and get fit. Bicycling is for anyone that is willing to take the time and do what they need to do to have a better body.

In fact, it is one of the best outdoor aerobic exercises that you can do without having to go through a lot of changes. If you want a healthier cardiovascular system, bicycling will do the trick. It also

Aerobic Exercise: Great Routines to Foster Healthy Living
strengthens your legs as the pedals go up and down while you're riding.

If you are one of those who has a bicycle but has not used it in a while, crank it up and get into shape. Using elbow grease to lubricate it, you will be able to take it on a spin. Some people say that bicycling is better than walking.

It depends on how you feel about each aerobic exercise. Plus, bicycling is another exercise where you won't have to come out of your pocket a lot. As you are getting your workout in, you are also helping the environment by not adding to the pollution that is already there.

Just remember to take your time when you first start out and gradually increase when you are ready. Before you know it, you will start to look fit and buff.

Chapter 17- A Few Tips To Remember

Before any form of exercise is done, a doctor should be consulted.

Consult with your physician before starting any aerobic exercise program.

Once you get the all clear, start off with aerobic exercises at least three times a week and work your way up.

Work to increase your heart rate so that you get more oxygen to breathe. Also, your blood will start flowing properly.

Stick to realistic goals during your journey of getting fit.

CONCLUSION

No matter what kind of aerobic exercise you get into, it's important to stick with it. You must be consistent for however many days you are committed each week. It's important to stay committed because you will eventually see results.

Don't look for that quick fix where you can lose so weight quickly. Take your time and allow it to come off on its own. When you start out fast, you can risk injuring yourself, which will slow things down.

Don't be in a hurry to start the first one you see. Evaluate yourself and know what you can and cannot do. Once you keep at it, you will see results that you will approve of.

Jana Duncan

RESOURCES

http://www.ehow.com/how-does_4574009_aerobic-exercise-work.html

http://www.ehow.com/about_4740202_step-aerobics.html

http://www.ehow.com/how_2287286_have-proper-technique-step-aerobics.html

http://www.ehow.com/topic_2076_aerobic-steps-basics.html

http://running.about.com/lr/get_started_with_running/347876/4/

http://running.about.com/od/getstartedwithrunning/tp/startarunninghabit.htm

http://running.about.com/od/nutritionandhydration/a/hydration101.htm

http://running.about.com/od/getstartedwithrunning/tp/startarunninghabit.htm

http://running.about.com/od/howtorun/tp/runningform.htm

http://running.about.com/od/faqsforbeginners/f/avoidbounce.htm

http://www.ehow.com/how_5362557_make-walking-aerobic-exercise.html

http://www.ehow.com/how_5356674_fit-walking-day.html

Aerobic Exercise: Great Routines to Foster Healthy Living
http://www.ehow.com/how_5550953_enjoy-walking-workout.html

http://bicycling.about.com/od/trainingandfitness/a/better_body.htm

http://www.coolbiking.com/blog/health-fitness/exercise/how-to-get-fit-and-keep-fit-by-cycling-for-fitness/

http://en.wikipedia.org/wiki/Cycling

ABOUT THE AUTHOR

I'm passionate about working out and coming up with new workout routines; especially for aerobics as it's such a full-body workout and so good for you. I've been doing this for quite some years and don't see myself stopping any time soon. It truly has been a way of life for me. Although I have an extremely busy schedule, I find a way to get it done.

A lot of what I encourage in my books is how to set exercise goals that you can be comfortable with and actually achieve without getting too flustered. There is something that can be designed for everyone depending on their specific needs. I've found mine and helping others to find theirs is what I set out to do.

My children are teenagers now and although I put no pressure on them to workout as I do, I set an example and am pleased to see how much they respect what I do and how they are so much more conscientious of their health as they continue to develop.